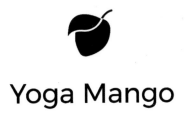

Yoga Mango

GENERAL LOWER BACK WITH NECK, SHOULDERS AND HIP FOCUS

Yoga Back Helper Minis

By Christine Pitt

Yoga Therapist (PG Dip IYT),

Yoga Alliance Professionals Senior Yoga Teacher,

Yoga Alliance Professionals Certified Trainer,

British Wheel of Yoga Teacher,

BCYT Accredited (British Council for Yoga Therapy)

CNHC Registered

'You're as Young as Your Spine is Flexible'

Chinese Proverb

TABLE OF CONTENTS

BACK HELPER SERIES: GENERAL LOWER BACK WITH NECK, SHOULDERS AND HIP FOCUS

AIM
To give you some simple back helpers within reach of anyone. You will have some easy-to-remember tools at your fingertips to relieve back strain or pain and feel calm and relaxed. You don't have to have practised yoga to benefit from these simple, gentle and very effective movements that are accessible to everybody.

We do not see the world as it is: we see it as we are.

The Talmund

BACK INTRODUCTION
Keep moving! Use it or lose it! The spine needs movement to lubricate the joints and provide nutrition to the spongey discs between the vertebrae. The natural spinal curves can become imbalanced by poor posture, injury or repetitive movement. The spinal column is a series of curves defined by the shape of the vertebrae ad the shape of the intervertebral discs and supporting ligaments. The thoracic (upper back) and sacral (pelvic) convex curves are the first to develop. Later in crawling and standing, the cervical (neck) and lumbar (lower back) concave curvatures develop as children learn to lift their heads and then to stand. The curves are designed to absorb shock and facilitate the full range of movement throughout the spinal column. These curves due to a variety of reasons, poor posture, injury, repetitive movement, stress even can become imbalanced and pain can arise from simply lifting something heavy or doing an everyday activity like gardening.

BENEFITS OF YOGA FOR NECK, SHOULDERS AND HIPS

Yoga restores flexibility, improves circulation to the joints and facilitates the release of endorphins, the body's own natural pain-killers, brings relief from tension and stress in the body. The aim is to calm inflammation, open the joints and encourage blood and fluid flow which in turn allows more comfortable movement in the area.

Can help to:

Relieve back pain

Reduce stress

Improves breathing

Increases flexibility

Improves posture

Engages abdominal muscles for core strength

HOW DO THE NECK, SHOULDERS AND HIPS RELATE TO THE BACK

Yoga affects not only the spine but corrects musculoskeletal imbalances anywhere in the body. No back problem can be isolated, the whole body is involved. Many factors may contribute to a bad back: tight or weak muscles, poor postures, obesity, emotional stress and a lack of full movement range in the peripheral joints, the shoulders and the hips. The neck is an extension of the spine.

As we age, ligaments and tendons can shorten fractionally. Even if we are active, sports like tennis, golf or cricket tend to involve asymmetrical movement where we tend to favour one side as we move. The range of motion of certain joints decreases. Discs lose their ability to absorb shock, muscles weaken and bones can lose mass. If we add in a sedentary lifestyle where we spend time sitting perhaps in cars, at our desks, in front of the television and potentially poor posture or slouching, this can add to our back problems. The lower back is particularly prone to disc herniation and disc degeneration problems because it's a weight-bearing junction linking the pelvis and spine. Help is at hand because yoga is one of the best ways to keep the back pain-free and healthy.

HYPER-MOBILE INSTABILITY AND SLIPPING/DISLOCATION

Sometimes joints can have too much movement and this can lead to instability and in extreme cases, dislocation. Post-pregnancy when the muscles have been stretched and are still soft can also lead to slight instability and in some cases, slipping or dislocation. Strength and alignment are key to protection.

TIGHTNESS AND RESTRICTED MOVEMENT

Abdominal strengthening is commonly recommended for back health. To protect the back from injury, we should do more than core-strengthening exercises. No back problem can be isolated from the rest of the body. To protect the back from injury and maintain back health, whole body movements, designed to integrate and benefit the entire body, are most beneficial. Yoga postures lengthen connective tissue, expand range of movement, improve posture and protect against back injury.

Other aspects of back issues include for example, tight hamstrings (because they can pull the pelvis out of alignment). Also, tight hip flexors in front of the thigh (iliopsoas and quadriceps) can cause issues and pain because the iliopsoas links into the lumbar vertebrae. Other muscles supporting the spine can also become tight so relaxation and releasing these is important (quadratus lumborum in the lower back; the erector spinae along the spine). The piriformis muscle, a hip rotator, deep in the buttocks, can also be tight (and can cause pain – sciatica).

The whole-body yoga approach balances not just the spine but imbalances elsewhere in the rest of the body bringing pain-relief and natural body alignment.

You are in the present moment: there is no judgement. Be kind to yourself, accept any limitations – just be!

ANTI-INFLAMMATORY BOOST

Nature's anti-inflammatories such as ginger or turmeric (curcumin) can help. A slice of ginger in hot water, maybe with some lemon as a drink first thing in the morning or anytime during the day, even before bed. Yoga is naturally anti-inflammatory with its gentle movement, designed to calm and soothe.

Dr Elizabeth Blackburn and Dr Elissa Epel examine how we can slow the way we age at a fundamental level in their book, *The Telomere Effect*. This includes looking at 'the wonder of yoga', 'known to be excellent for holding back the ravages of time on the body' and 'proven not only to improve your mood but also to reduce blood pressure and possibly even quell damaging levels of inflammation in the body'. Recently it was also shown to increase the bone density of the spine if practised long-term.

GENERAL MOVEMENT GUIDE FOR THE BACK IN RELATION TO THE NECK, SHOULDERS AND HIPS

Postural and alignment awareness – no slouching! Sometimes joints can be very mobile or hyper-mobile and this can lead to joints slipping out of alignment fractionally. Over-stretched ligaments, weak supporting muscles and potentially decreasing spinal disc spaces (this can be exacerbated from lack of spinal movement) can all play their part. Focus on alignment and postural awareness for strength together with mindful awareness of movement.

Balanced body and joint movement for mobility and lubrication - move carefully and with attention.

Focus on breathing and relaxation. These relax the muscles promoting better blood flow and circulation to the joints by altering the sympathetic/parasympathetic nerve signal to relax.

For everyday life and movement, pay attention and move with awareness, no sudden or sharp movement!

A note on the 'core' for stabilising movement. If you make a sudden movement, as you might do in sporting activities, you can fractionally engage your lower abdomen towards your spine, like zipping up a pair of jeans, lifting up and in, also slightly lifting the perineum up (and you may find you engage the entire lower area and clench your buttocks as it can be difficult to separate muscles out. This is fine too) Engaging your 'core' protects your lower back as your back is not having to do all the work. You can also enhance this effect by breathing out or exhaling as you make the movement. Whatever works for you.

YOGA MANGO CASE STUDIES

Brenda had sciatica, a pain from her lower back along the back of her leg. She also plays golf. She initially came for a lower back rehabilitation programme but has carried on ever since. Gentle yoga for the lower back keeps her mobile, she adapts what she's learned to her golf and everyday activities and says that she 'feels so much better, more mobile and that her son thinks her posture has improved since she's been coming to yoga.'

Babs broke her hip, she tripped over, carrying some books, in the hospital where she worked. She recovered very well but was understandably apprehensive about hip movement and being 'safe'. We started with gentle movements, getting the circulation moving within the hip area. Simple yoga, adapted for individual needs, any time, any place. A toolkit not just for regaining flexibility but Babs also says 'it gave her confidence to move safely' and like a lot of people, she says 'she feels so much better' afterwards.

Lindsay has a tumour at the base of her spine. We adapt any restful positions with soft support and Lindsay is able to enjoy yoga, using some simple modifications and support. She always says she's a lot calmer and 'less stressed' after coming to yoga.

Margaret tends to be breathless as well as having lower back issues. She can't get onto the floor but enjoys yoga with individual modifications. She rests in a seated position, with support. Focus on co-ordinating movement with the breath is helpful and she feels 'more in control' and 'hopeful' as well as enjoying the yoga movement.

Owen is bent over. It's impossible to ask him to stand up straight but he can lift up slightly at his chest. This aligns his posture and gives his normally compressed organs a little more space.

Yoga really is for anyone, anytime, anywhere!

THE BODY SCAN OR 3-MINUTE BREATHING SPACE

Instant Calm! There are many ways to relax. Sometimes though this is easier said than done. A quick, mindful way to relax is applying ancient wisdom to today's modern stresses. Calming the mind and relaxing the body brings many benefits including the back as this helps to bring more nutrients via the blood as the muscles begin to release as well as optimal blood flow to help elimination of toxins from the system.

Seated or lying – be comfortable. Anywhere, any place, on its own or combined with other practices.

Mentally working your way up the body, drawing awareness to each part (it is not necessary to move any parts). Your own special areas or specific parts can be added or left, entirely according to your own preferences and needs. This is a suggested sequence you can adapt for yourself.

Become aware of:

Toes and feet

Heels, ankles

Lower legs, shins, calves

Knees and backs of the knees

Thighs

Pelvis and hips

Abdomen, stomach

Chest, breastbone

Collar bones, across shoulders to the upper arms

Elbows, forearms, through to the wrists, hands, back of the hands, palms of the hands, thumbs and fingers- first finger, second finger, third finger, fourth finger and little finger

Back to the buttocks, up the long muscles either side of the back, lower back, mid-back, shoulder blades, between the shoulder blades, upper back, across the shoulders to the neck, back of the head, ears, top of the head, over the forehead, across the eyebrows, between the eyebrows, around the eyes, the ears, between the ears, down the nose, across the cheeks, around the lips, teeth and gums, along the jawline, chin, down to the base of the throat, the whole body, the whole body, the whole body.

Allow the breath to flow, through the nostrils, cool as the breath flows in, warm and soft as the breath flows out.

Take a deep breath, sigh the breath away and open your eyes.

This is just one of many variations of a body scan. By bringing your attention to each body part, however briefly, you are diverting attention to that part and this adds as a mini-distraction, slowing your breath, putting in a pause.

Stop! Brings moment-to-moment awareness that can enable a new perspective of choice and possibility rather than operating from normal habit. You become aware of your body and your breath. The quality of breath directly reflects you, your body, your health and your clarity of mind.

GENERAL PRACTICES FOR THE BACK LEARNING TO RELIEVE AND MANAGE BACK PAIN, SOOTHE AND CALM THE BODY AND MIND

WHO

For anyone, anywhere, anytime.

WHY

The sequences here are all designed to soothe your back and are suitable for many back conditions. Work to where you feel comfortable, moving as little or as much as is good for you.

USE IT OR LOSE IT

Your own back needs are like choosing your own shade of colour from the palette.

The back is meant to be moved in a number of directions for optimal back health but like colour, different shades suit different people.

Anyone who has back movement restriction or pain, benefits from relaxing, focusing on the breath and making very gentle and safe movement. Lack of back movement can lead to stiffness and inflexibility. This should feel comfortable, calming and relaxing as well as improving flexibility.

EVERYONE IS DIFFERENT

Learn to expect the unexpected. No two people are the same and their movement requirements, even for the same condition, can vary hugely. You can have, in the same class, someone who can't kneel, someone who doesn't like standing and someone who doesn't like sitting!

BREATHE

Co-ordinate your movement with your breath. Inhale as you stretch your toes up for example and exhale as you point your toes down. This has the effect of slowing your breath down, relaxing your body and mind. There are many breathing exercises you can explore in yoga.

FOR HOW LONG

Anybody with any back condition including stiff neck, shoulders and hips should be able to find something here that suits them. Work to your own limit. There is no quick fix but gentle and safe stability with confidence. This is no competition. The programmes are designed for you to get the most out of them and that means working to where you feel comfortable and taking responsibility for your back. Anybody can do yoga, even lying in bed!

Choose a sequence that's best for you.

The 'dynamic' poses where you move in/out you may want to practise 3-6 times or for however many times feel appropriate. The more restful poses you can practise for up to 10-20 breaths or again longer if this feels relaxing. The sequences aren't very long, 10-15 minutes, depending on how long you feel like staying in the poses. If you are resting you may want to spend 10-15 minutes or longer just in one pose. Resting and relaxing gives your body an opportunity to release any tightness.

You are in the present moment: there is no judgement. Be kind to yourself, accept any limitations – just be!

YOGA SEQUENCES

SEATED YOGA FOR EVERYONE (BACK, NECK, SHOULDERS AND HIPS): JOINT MOVEMENT

STANDING YOGA FOR EVERYONE: EXPLORING BACK MOVEMENT WITH POSTURAL AWARENESS

LYING YOGA FOR EVERYONE: LOWER BACK PAIN RELIEF PRACTICE

MIXED LYING/STANDING YOGA FOR EVERYONE (BACK, NECK, SHOULDERS AND HIPS): WITH POSTURAL AWARENESS AND ABDOMINAL FOCUS

REST OR EMERGENCY POSES FOR BACK RELIEF FOR EVERYONE

LYING PRACTICE FOR BACK, NECK, SHOULDERS AND HIPS

Choose a practice that suits you. If you prefer to stay seated or there is no opportunity to stand, for example, choose the seated yoga for everyone. All the practices are safe and gentle.

SEATED YOGA FOR EVERYONE (BACK, NECK, SHOULDERS AND HIPS):
JOINT MOVEMENT

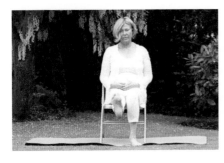

Feet: one foot at a time or both feet together, each movement to co-ordinate with breathing in/out. Each exercise 3-10 times.

Move toes up/down
Circle ankles in each direction
Stretch toes out; curl them in

Brings blood flow to the joints in the foot and ankle – the foundation of our posture, beginning to activate circulation and boosting our immune system.

Knees: holding under one knee, let the knee swing backwards and forwards. 3-5 times each side.

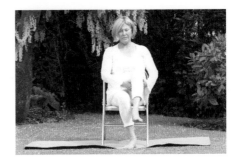

Bringing movement, circulation and lubrication to the knee joint.

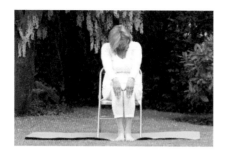

Sitting with hands on the knees: sit up as you breathe in; round your back as you breathe out. 3-10 times (if this feels releasing, you can practise up to 25 times or even more!)

Warming the spine, bringing gentle movement to the vertebrae. Move as little or as much as you like. The movement is controlled with your hands on your knees.

Holding either your knees or the sides of the chair, inhaling as you extend one arm to the side and up. Exhale as you bring the arm down. 2-3 times each side.
A lateral stretch to the spine. Lengthening along the side, creating space for your internal organs, helping with your lung capacity. Your arms can be bent or straight.

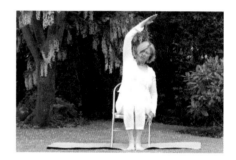

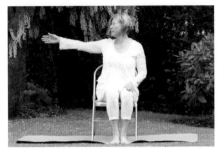

Hands on knees; inhale and open your right arm to the side, following your hand movement with your eyes. You move as little or as far as feels good. Exhale as you bring your arm back, placing your hand on your knee. 1-2 times each side.

Starting to explore gentle rotation. This can be a few inches even. Rotation is re-aligning for the spine and is one of the directions the spine needs to move for optimal health but caution for some spinal conditions, less is more. Be guided by how you feel.

Hands on your knees; breathe in and sit up, lengthening along the spine, come slightly forward. Breathe for 3-5 breaths. You can optionally use a bolster/cushion/pillow to place on your lap for support with hands either on the bolster or elbows on the bolster, hands supporting head.

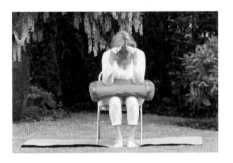

Releasing for the lower back, to within your own limits: calming for the mind.

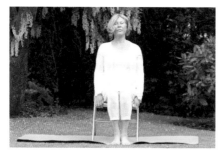

Sitting up and either holding your knees or holding the edge of the chair, lift at the sternum or chest area. You can look slightly upwards being careful with putting your head too far back). Breathe here for 3-5 breaths.

This very gentle backbend movement balances the previous forward movement of the spine, lengthening the body and creating space for your internal organs, space for your lungs.

Sitting up, place your hands on your knees, come gently forwards again, for 3-5 breaths

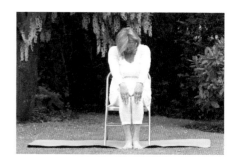

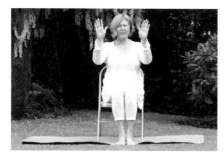

Hands: you can move both hands together (one at a time is fine too). Co-ordinate your movement with your breath, inhaling as point your hands/fingers upwards, breathing out as you move them down. Each exercise 3-10 times.

Move hands up/down
Circle wrists in each direction
Stretch fingers out; curl them in

Hands are an extension of the heart and these simple movements activate circulation and bring blood to the wrists and finger joints.

Sitting, place your hands, one over the other, at the heart level. Inhaling and open your hands out to the side; exhaling and bring your hands back to your heart. 3-5 times (or longer if you find this soothing).

A very gentle activation to the circulatory and respiratory functions. You can open your hands as much or as little as you like.

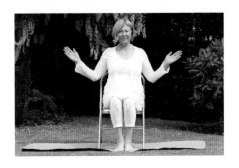

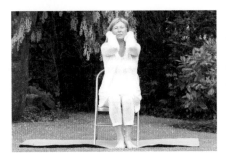

Placing your hands, finger tips at the top of your shoulders, inhale and stretch them out in front of you ; exhale and bring them back, touching your shoulders again.

3-5 times. A gentle shoulder movement.

Sitting, hands relaxed, inhale and turn your head towards the right, exhale and bring your head back to centre. Repeat to the other side, 3-5 times each side moving your neck as little or as much as feels comfortable.

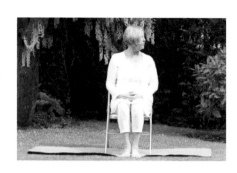

Gentle neck movement. You can optionally also gently move your chin slightly downwards as you move from side to side. This slightly elongates the muscles along the back of your neck that can get tight.

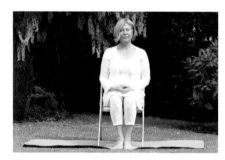

Sit comfortably, hands resting in your lap and breathe.

You can just become aware of your breath coming in as your abdomen slightly extends and breathing out as your abdomen moves back towards the spine. You are breathing in/out through your nose. You can count 1234 as you breathe in and 1234 as you breathe out or just close your eyes and relax. You can stay here for 10-20 breaths or longer.

You can optionally start with exercise by saying 'haa' to yourself as you breathe out - in this case you are exhaling through your mouth rather than your nose. This adds a very gentle abdominal engagement for a few breaths. Then breathe in/out through your nose as you spend the next few breaths relaxing.

STANDING YOGA FOR EVERYONE: EXPLORING BACK MOVEMENT WITH POSTURAL AWARENESS

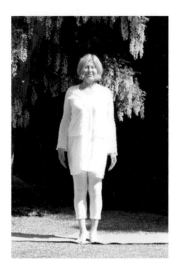

This entire sequence can be practised from 1-3-10 times, according to how you feel and time available to you.

Stand, feet firmly into the ground as if you're pushing the earth away from you. Feet can be hip-width apart for a sense of feeling grounded. Lift and roll your shoulders back. Imagine lifting your sternum, the centre of your chest fractionally upwards. Relax. Postural awareness.

Inhale and lift your arms sideways and upwards. Go only as high as feels comfortable. This can be to shoulder level or the full pose, hands above your head. If your head starts to come forward, you've come too far. Clasp your hands together and reverse them upwards. Inhale and lengthen your body upwards.

Stretching further, the sequence begins to warm up the spine. The sequence can gently decompress the segments promoting increased circulation to the spinal discs.

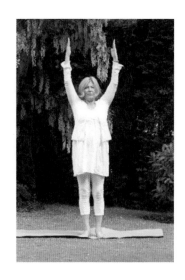

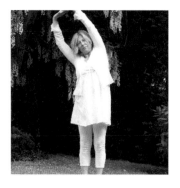

Exhale and move slightly to the right; inhale to centre; exhale move slightly to the left. Lateral movement side-to-side

Return to inhaling and lengthening the spine; exhale and rotate or turn slightly to one side; inhale to the centre and exhale, turning to the other side.

A very gentle rotation, entirely within your control as you can move as little or as much as feels appropriate – or not at all, you can keep this movement as optional.

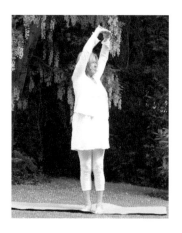

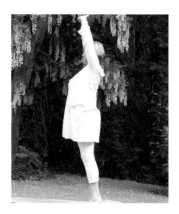

Inhaling and rise onto your toes, looking ahead. Stay for 1-3-5 breaths.

A balance, bringing focus, steadying for the mind and inviting left-right brain co-ordination.

Exhaling, lower your arms

extending them to shoulder height. Look beyond the third finger of one hand as you exhale; inhale to centre; exhale to the other side, looking beyond the third finger.
Gentle neck movement

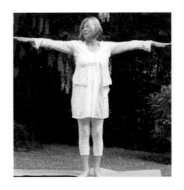

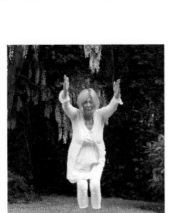

Inhale, raising your hands above your head once more, or as high as feels comfortable, feet hip-width apart. Exhale, bending your knees, inhale come to standing.

Bending your knees engages your abdominal muscles. You can have your hands at shoulder-height or even on the waist as a modification.

Come to standing, lift and roll your shoulders back.

Awareness of standing encourages postural alignment.

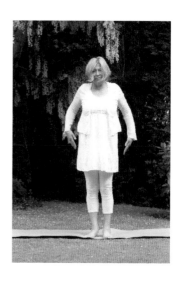

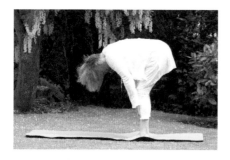

Placing your hands on your thighs for support, exhale and bend your knees, rolling forward, as little or as much as you feel comfortable with. You have the option of placing your hands on the shins if you come forward more or even placing the hands on the floor.

Coming forward is calming, how far you come forward is up to you.

Wherever your hands are, inhale, press with your hands into your legs and lengthen along the spine by raising the back of the head slightly whilst still looking down along the floor. Exhale and come back to your forward position, the elbows can move out to the side.

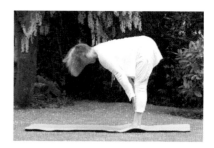

Extending your spine is giving space to the vertebrae with the support of your hands.

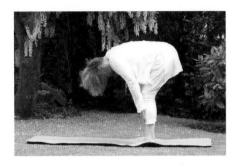

Inhale, you can use your hands as support, to roll up, vertebra by vertebra, to standing. Lift and roll your shoulders.

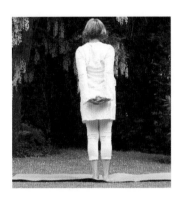

Clasp your hands behind your back, aiming the knuckles towards the floor.

You can clasp your wrists as a modification. If this is difficult, simply lift and roll your shoulders, standing up straight.

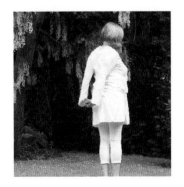

Exhale and turn slightly to one side, inhale to centre and exhale, turn slightly to the other side, inhale to centre.

Release the hands, stand up tall, inhale and raise your hands sideways.

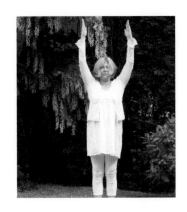

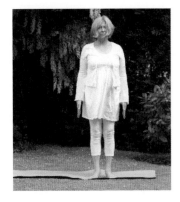

Exhale and lower your hands.

LYING YOGA FOR EVERYONE: LOWER BACK PAIN RELIEF PRACTICE

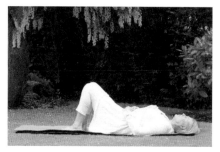

Come to lying; feet on the floor, hip-width apart, hands resting on the abdomen and become aware quite simply of your breath. There is nothing for you to do, just notice your breath coming in, expanding the abdomen slightly and breathing out, the abdomen moves away from your hands. Stay for up to 6 breaths (1 breath = 1 inhale and 1 exhale)

If you have one side that is slightly more painful than the other, start by hugging your 'good' side into your chest. Again stay for up to 6 breaths.

Switch sides and hug the other 'bad' side in towards your chest. Stay for up to 6 breaths or fractionally longer on this 'bad' side.

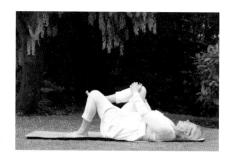

Just enjoy the gently stretch. The back muscles are not being asked to support you in this semi-supine position and can begin to 'relax' and let go.

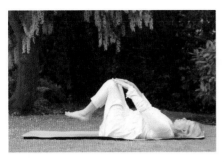

Now hug both knees into the chest, for up to 6 breaths.

Semi-supine positions are releasing and relaxing for the lower back.

Come back to placing both feet on the floor, hands on the abdomen, for up to 6 breaths
Rest

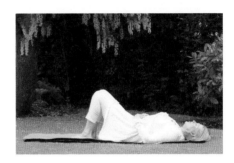

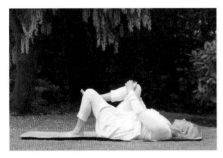

Hug one knee into the chest as you exhale, still holding the knee, inhale and relax the knee a few inches away from you. Repeat this movement for a total of up to 6 times.
Change sides.

Releasing and pain-relieving.

Hug both knees into the chest whilst holding them and release them away as you inhale, up to a total of 6 times

Releasing and pain-relieving.

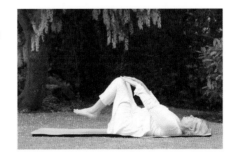

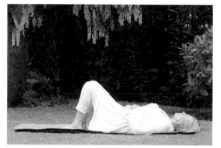

Release both feet to the floor and either relax with hands on the abdomen, or come to lying with any support you might like (under the head; under the knees; under the feet or a combination of these) and relax for up to 6- 10-20 breaths or for however long feels comfortable.

Relax and rest.

MIXED LYING/STANDING YOGA FOR EVERYONE (BACK, NECK, SHOULDERS AND HIPS): WITH POSTURAL AWARENESS AND ABDOMINAL FOCUS

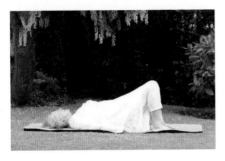

Pelvic Tilt:
Exhale and flatten the lower back towards the floor, inhale and release.

Massages the lower back and activates movement in the lower abdomen. Helps to increase lower back flexibility, massaging the lower back area, increasing circulation. 5-10 times (up to 20-25 times) depending on how you feel.

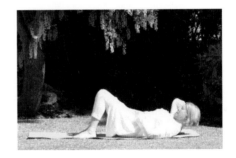

Yoga Sit Ups:
Knees bent, one hand on abdomen, the other behind the head, supporting the neck and exhaling lift the head a few inches off the ground. This engages the lower abdominal muscles (your core) without straining the neck. If your abdomen starts to dome, you've gone too far! Lifting the head is also optional! 3 times each side.

Engaging the abdominal muscles can take the strain away from the back muscles doing all the work. Here on the floor, the back muscles are supported and you can focus solely on the abdominals.

Windscreen Wipers:
Let your knees move a few inches to one side as you breathe out; inhale to the centre and exhale as you move your knees to the other side. The wider you have your feet, the easier you will find this. Find where you are comfortable. The hips can lift off the floor. You can move a few inches or the knees can touch the floor.

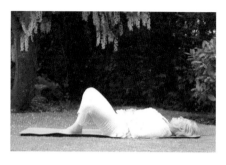

You can gently engage your pelvic floor and slightly contract or engage your lower abdomen. 3-10 times to either side. It's up to you. Hug your knees into your chest, roll to your right side and come to standing.

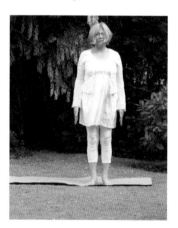

Mountain Pose:
Roll to the right and come to standing. Press your feet into the floor or have a sense of pressing the earth away from you; everything below your navel is heavy, going towards the floor and everything above your navel is light, rising up in the air. This gives you a sense of balance in your posture. Lift at your sternum, your chest level fractionally. Lift and roll your shoulders back. Turn your head from side to side.

You are balanced in your standing posture. Lift and roll one shoulder forward; then backward and then roll the other shoulder. Turn your head again, slowly, from side to side and back to the centre. Inhale and raise your hands, palms facing inwards. Exhale and lower your hands, bending your knees and rolling down to the floor once again.

Knee to Chest:

Lying, hug one knee into your chest. You can rock from side to side, massaging along the lower back/sacral area. You can gently extend the leg upwards, holding underneath to extend your hamstrings. Hug back into the chest and change sides.

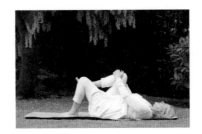

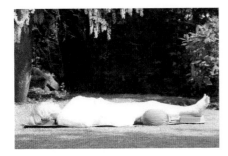

Relax:

This can either be on your back, with support possibly under your head, under your knees and can be under your feet. On your back with knees bent. Or over a bolster, in Child's Pose. For 10-20 breaths or for however long feels good for you.

REST OR EMERGENCY POSES FOR BACK RELIEF FOR EVERYONE

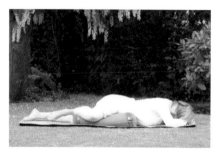

Recovery Position:
Use support under the bent leg on the side that is painful.

Lower back pain relief. Stay for as long as is comfortable.

Using a chair or equivalent, for this semi-supine resting position as an alternative. You could rest your legs up the wall too, feet against the wall, using support.

Lower back pain relief. Stay for as long as is comfortable.

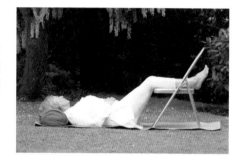

MIXED LYING/STANDING YOGA FOR NECK, SHOULDERS AND HIPS: WITH POSTURAL AWARENESS AND ABDOMINAL FOCUS

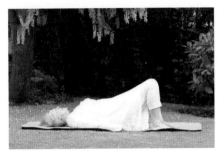

Pelvic Tilt:
Exhale and flatten the lower back towards the floor, inhale and release. Massages the lower back and activates movement in the lower abdomen. Helps to increase lower back flexibility, massaging the lower back area, increasing circulation. 5-10 times (up to 20-25 times) depending on how you feel.

Yoga Sit Ups:
Knees bent, one hand on abdomen, the other behind the head, supporting the neck and exhaling lift the head a few inches off the ground. This engages the lower abdominal muscles (your core) without straining the neck. If your abdomen starts to dome, you've gone too far! Lifting the head is also optional!   3 times each side.

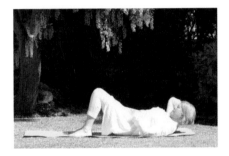

Engaging the abdominal muscles can take the strain away from the back muscles doing all the work. Here on the floor, the back muscles are supported and you can focus solely on the abdominals.

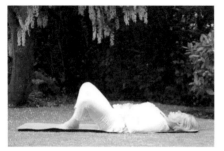

Windscreen Wipers:
Let your knees move a few inches to one side as you breathe out; inhale to the centre and exhale as you move your knees to the other side. The wider you have your feet, the easier you will find this. Find where you are comfortable. The hips can lift off the floor. You can move a few inches or the knees can touch the floor. You can gently engage your pelvic floor and slightly contract or engage your lower abdomen. 3-10 times to either side. It's up to you. Hug your knees into your chest, roll to your right side and come to standing.

Standing Mountain Pose:
Roll to the right and come to standing. Press your feet into the floor or have a sense of pressing the earth away from you; everything below your navel is heavy, going towards the floor and everything above your navel is light, rising up in the air. This gives you a sense of balance in your posture. Lift at your sternum, your chest level fractionally. Lift and roll your shoulders back.

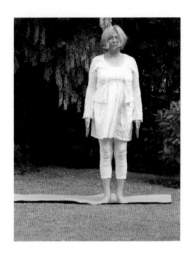

Neck:
Turn your head from side to side. You are balanced in your standing posture. Exhale as you turn your head; inhale as you come back to centre.

Slightly dip your chin, lengthening the back of your neck as you turn your head to one side; return your head to centre and exhale to the other side.

Shoulders:
Lift and roll one shoulder forward; then backward and then roll the other shoulder. You could also simply shrug one shoulder at a time, lifting as you inhale and letting the shoulder drop as you exhale.

Turn your head again, slowly, from side to side and back to the centre.

Placing your fingertips on your collar bone, inhale and extend your arms, exhale and bring your fingers back to your collar bone. 3-6 times.

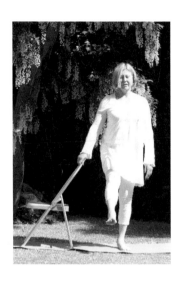

Standing Mountain Pose

Hips:
You can optionally hold a chair or wall for balance as you swing your leg to/fro.

Knee to Chest:
Lying, hug one knee into your chest. You can rock from side to side, massaging along the lower back/sacral area. You can gently extend the leg upwards, holding underneath to extend your hamstrings. Hug back into the chest and change sides.

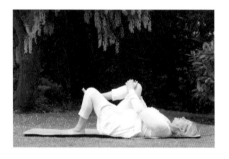

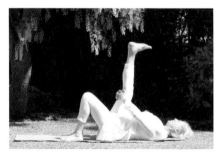

Holding the leg underneath, stretch your leg upwards, extending your heel. The leg can remain bent at the knee. This is a gentle hamstring stretch along the back of the leg.

Hips:

'Threading the Needle' pose begins to open up the hip in a gentle external rotation. You will also feel this at the outer hip level on one side. Stay here for up to 6 breaths.

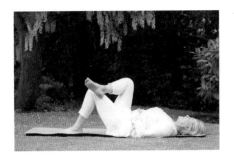

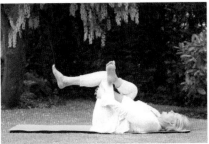

Briefly hug knees to chest.

This version of 'Threading the Needle' pose is slightly stronger. If this is too much, return to the previous pose. Stay here for 3-6 breaths.

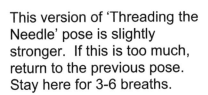

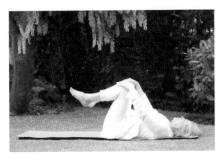

Whilst still holding both knees, open knees slightly to form a V. Make small circles in one direction, you are 'lubricating' the hip joint. 3-6 times. Reverse your circle, moving in the opposite direction (clockwise and anti-clockwise).

Lying Tree:
Open one side, foot against the other leg, you can use support under your bent leg for your thigh/knee. This is opening for the hips. Change to the other side. Up to 6 breaths or longer. You may also enjoy placing the soles of both feet together, again with support if you need it.

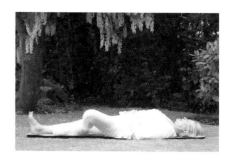

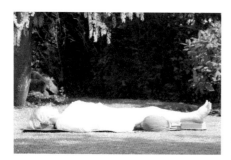

Relax:
This can either be on your back, with support possibly under your head, under your knees and can be under your feet. On your back with knees bent. Or over a bolster, in Child's Pose. For 10-20 breaths or for however long feels good for you.

About Christine

Christine is a yoga therapist (PG Dip IYT) with additional specialist training in backs, Ayurveda and Mindfulness. She is CNHC registered and accredited by The British Council for Yoga Therapy. She is a Yoga Alliance Professionals Senior Teacher, a Yoga Alliance Professionals Certified Trainer and a British Wheel of Yoga Teacher. She is also a registered teacher for the Lower Healthy Backs Programme, a trained teacher of Yoga for Cancer, a Reiki Teacher and Oriental Remedial Therapist.

She's also experienced pain!

She incorporates her journey of learning that has taken her on many paths with different teachers and yoga traditions into her yoga therapy training.

Upcoming Yoga Back Helper Minis

Christine has written a series of yoga back helper books. Further information will be available via www.yogamango.com. These include:

- Arthritis
- Herniated Disc and Pinched Nerve
- Neck, Shoulders and Hips
- Osteoporosis
- Pregnancy and Post-Natal Lower Back Health
- Sciatica
- Scoliosis
- Yoga Back Care for Sports

With grateful thanks to Dr Jan Maneira and Dr Charlotte Keywood for their help and endorsement of all material contained in the Yoga Back Helper Minis series.

In addition, grateful thanks to Karen Morton, Consultant Obstetrician and Gynaecologist, for her endorsement in respect of Yoga Back Helper Minis: Pregnancy and Post-Natal Lower Back Health.

'I have carefully reviewed this work and can wholeheartedly endorse the potential benefits of this approach to a multitude of health problems.'

Stay in Touch

Christine is very happy to answer any questions you may have from this training workshop or for any students coming to your class with back issues.

Details about further workshops and training including Back Care; Yoga Therapy and Ayurveda plus a 200-hour Yoga with a Therapy Focus training can be found on:

www.yogamango.com

Yoga Mango can also be found on Facebook: Yoga Mango and Yoga Mango Therapy.

You can also contact Christine via e-mail: christinetms@aol.com and contact@yogamango.com

Printed in Great Britain
by Amazon